I0429413

AUTOIMMUNE COOKBOOK

The Natural Autoimmune Disease Solution - Complete
Starter's Guide

All Rights Reserved. No part of this publication may be reproduced in any form or by any means, including scanning, photocopying, or otherwise without prior written permission of the copyright holder. Copyright © 2014

Table of Contents

Introduction

Feeling symptoms that might be associated to an underlying medical condition is a very uncomfortable feeling. Some individuals, however, manifest more anxiety than others. If you experience fatigue, fever, headaches or malaise and you react as though you have some dreaded disease, you will probably be accused of being a hypochondriac - one who is excessively preoccupied and unreasonably fearful of having a serious affliction that does not even exist. Even if rashes and painful joints are added to the previously mentioned four symptoms, one can not just break into hysteria about having an autoimmune disease.

While it is true that fatigue, fever, headaches, malaise, rashes and painful joints are some of the more common symptoms of an autoimmune disease, these conditions are present in a host of other non-autoimmune afflictions. Nevertheless, about 7 out of 10 patients subsequently diagnosed with an autoimmune disease have unfortunately been thought to be suffering from hypochondria in the earlier stages of their illness. This was bared by the American Autoimmune Related Diseases Association (AARDA). Do you think that it is possible to observe some symptoms that could possibly be clues that you might have an autoimmune disease early on? For starters, autoimmune diseases can be difficult to diagnose early in the course of the disease.

There are a lot of obstacles that may hinder earlier diagnosis of an autoimmune disease. Results of laboratory tests are inadequate to confirm a diagnosis. Anecdotal records of many patients also indicate that most autoimmune diseases either flare up (i.e., symptoms tend to worsen) or go into remission for a period of time. Remission is the tendency of some symptoms to disappear temporarily, only to reappear at some point in time. Whatever these symptoms are, they pose a challenge not only to the patient but to the physician monitoring the condition as well. Often, a patient may need to be referred from one specialist to another for about five or more years until a diagnosis of an autoimmune disease can be confirmed with certainty.

It is a common thing among people with autoimmune diseases to complain or be very frustrated about being required by their physician to return for follow-up sessions without being told what their ailment is in the early course of the disease. Other patients say that their symptoms are short-lived and their laboratory tests are inconclusive earlier on and had been previously told that their symptoms are nothing of a serious nature. Others are not quite impressed that their physicians can only manage the consequences of inflammation brought about by the autoimmune disease. Doctors specializing in lupus and rheumatoid arthritis report that some of their patients respond to medication that slow or stop the immune system's damaging rampage on the kidney and joints, respectively. However, nothing has come up that can generally suppress the immune system's defective function.

The Enigma of Autoimmune Diseases

It is quite interesting to know what autoimmune diseases really are, but sadly, this is just about what is known. Why this type of diseases is on the rise during the last half century still baffles scientists despite significant advances in the field in terms of knowledge and technology. These diseases are not only difficult to diagnose but often turn up to be chronic illnesses. Graves' disease, hemolytic anemia, multiple sclerosis, myasthenia gravis, rheumatoid arthritis, type 1 diabetes, vasculitis, vitiligo, and a long list of other conditions are all autoimmune diseases.

An Inside Job

An autoimmune disease may be considered a crime perpetrated as an inside job. It is a disorder that results as your body's immune system, your natural defense against invading bacteria, viruses, toxins, cancerous cells, tissues and other harmful substances, mistakenly turns on your own body as an automatic response to what is it perceives as a threat to your health. Imagine your own protection system turning against you by some freak of nature. It knows every small detail of your body's natural immunity plan. Thus, it can easily breach whatever protection you have left for your own defense - an inside job!

It is easy for the body's natural antibodies to spot viruses, bacteria, and other organisms that invade our immune system because they are alien bodies. But when man's own protection against diseases goes haywire and attacks their own kind, the health consequences are staggering. How can you possibly introduce substances inside a person's body that will counteract the internal strife occurring among immune defenders to treat an autoimmune disease?

Not a Lost Cause

It is not, however, a lost cause yet. Reinforcement can be sent inside your body that your own immune system will not destroy. Your body needs food to survive. Food is nourishment and the faulty defenders of your immune system will not suspect food as a threat to your health. In other words, special nutrition can be utilized as an intervention to fortify your body's immune system.

The stronger your immune system is, the better chances you have in controlling the onslaught of the chronic symptoms of your specific autoimmune disorder. A good diet can, therefore, help reverse the effects of the disease. Carefully chosen nutrients can enter your body without opposition from the unsuspecting rebellious immune system cells and boost your immune system to a point that the healthy cells will multiply, outnumber, and destroy the disease cells that tend to turn against your body's own immune defenses.

People who have been diagnosed with autoimmune diseases receive treatment(s) that provide relief for the symptoms they experience. However, research has not found anything that would unlock the secret to turning off the immune response that attacks the body's own defenses against illnesses. Thus, to date, medical science is still continuously searching for that key knowledge that would stop the damage that an autoimmune disease causes to the body's natural security system for health and wellness.

Aside from being a chronic illness, an autoimmune disease requires lifelong care and monitoring even if the patient generally looks well or feels well. Only a few autoimmune diseases can be treated or cured to return the immune system to its normal function. The best that medical science can offer is management of the symptoms so that patients can deal with the pain, inflammation or other health conditions resulting from the body's autoimmune response.

The mystery of autoimmune disorders had not yet been unshrouded until this very day. No potent drug or vaccine had yet been synthesized in the world's most complex research facilities to destroy faulty defenders of your own immune system without adversely affecting normal and healthy cells. Nevertheless, the simplest kitchen can concoct yummy recipes that can heighten the efficiency of your immune system in neutralizing the flawed cells that triggered your autoimmune illness.

Nutrition to Strengthen the Immune System

Micronutrients support and revs up your immune system to help your body fight diseases. The following nutrients aid to boost your natural immunity from disease:

- Alkylglycerol
- Arginine
- Beta-carotene and carotenoids
- Beta glucan
- Choline
- Chromium
- Copper
- Dimethyglycine
- Essential fatty acids
- Folic Acid
- Glutamine
- Iron
- Manganese
- Phytonutrients
- Protein
- Selenium
- Vitamin A
- Vitamin B
- Vitamin C
- Vitamin E
- Zinc, etc.

This book's recipes were prepared with only the best foods that can help buttress your immune defenses against all kinds of illnesses, especially autoimmune diseases. Special emphasis is made to ensure that the autoimmune diet recipes do not provoke additional problems like the usual leaky gut condition that go with autoimmune ailments and trigger allergic reactions. The following food groups are known to be effective boosters of the immune system:

Anaerobic-Process Fermented Food

There are local grocers and supermarket chains that carry stocks of allergen-free fermented foods prepared via the anaerobic process. However, for better control of the ingredients, particularly sugar and additives, home-fermented foods are best:

- Coconut yogurt
- Fermented cucumber
- Kimchi
- Kombucha
- Pickled ginger
- Sauerkraut
- Water kefir

Coconut and its Derivatives

- Coconut butter
- Coconut cream
- Coconut oil
- Coconut flakes
- Coconut milk
- Coconut yogurt (without sugar)

Meats

If meat is permitted or allowed in limited amounts for your other medical conditions, then beef, chicken, fish can be included in the autoimmune diet. Lamb and turkey may also be used as ingredients. However, special precautions need to be observed:

- Fowl meat (chicken and turkey) and lamb should be free from antibiotics and hormones commonly found in grocery stores;
- Beef should also be sourced from antibiotic- and hormone-free, grass-fed and pastured cattle from a local farm. Organic meats are also acceptable.
- Refrain from choosing factory-farmed meats.

Organic Fruits with Low Glycemic Index

Fruits contain fructose, a natural sugar but also the sweetest of all sugars. Hence, not all fruits should find its way into the autoimmune diet. The following fruits are recommended for their low sugar content:

- Apple
- Apricot
- Avocado
- Berries
- Cherry
- Grapefruit
- Grapes
- Lemon
- Orange
- Peaches
- Pear
- Plum
- Prunes

Organic Vegetables

- Anise
- Artichoke
- Asparagus
- Beet green
- Bok choy
- Broccoli
- Cabbage
- Carrots
- Cauliflower
- Celery
- Chives
- Cucumber
- Garlic
- Kale
- Kohlrabi
- Leeks
- Lettuce
- Mustard greens
- Onion
- Radish
- Rhubarb
- Shallots
- Spinach
- Summer and winter squash
- Sweet potatoes
- Water chestnut
- Watercress
- Yam
- Zucchini

Spices

- Basil
- Balm (lemon balm)
- Bay leaf
- Black pepper
- Chamomile
- Chevril
- Cilantro
- Cinnamon or cassia
- Clove
- Coriander
- Dill
- Garlic
- Ginger
- Horseradish
- Lavender
- Lemongrass
- Mace
- Marjoram
- Mint
- Oregano
- Parsley
- Peppermint
- Rock salt (sea salt)
- Rosemary
- Saffron
- Sage
- Savory leaf
- Spearmint
- Tarragon
- Thyme
- Turmeric

The only noodle recommended for the autoimmune diet is the noodle made from shirataki yam. Soy- or tofu-based noodles are not to be included in the diet of autoimmune disease patients. Apple cider vinegar is recommended as substitute for the usual vinegar sold in the supermarket. Herbal tea, olives and olive oil are healthy fixtures of the autoimmune diet.

There are also supplements that medical science is looking into for their potential in boosting the immune system. Since these are supplements and not drugs, recipes for autoimmune diseases can be enriched with them. These promising supplements are:

- Aloe vera
- Astralagus membranes
- Echinacea
- Ginseng
- Licorice root
- Probiotics, etc.

If a person can be properly enlightened on how the body's own protection against diseases can be sustained and strengthened with the right kind and combination of natural foods, synthetic drugs and their inevitable side effects will no longer be needed. Come to think of it, there is more wisdom in defending your fortress from the inside than allowing an alien army to enter the fortress and fight the invaders from the outside. Your health is your fortress, and nutrition is a great way to strengthen your immune system against autoimmune diseases and other ailments in general. Fortifying your immune system is the best defense against illness. This book's recipes are specially prepared to help reverse the effects of autoimmune diseases in the most delicious way.

The Nightshade Vegetable Restriction

Vegetables that belong to the nightshade family can prove to be a problem for many people, especially those afflicted with autoimmune diseases. These include eggplants, tomatoes, hot and sweet peppers (except black pepper), and chili-based spices. Consumption of these vegetables should be shunned or minimized because of their saponin, lectin, and/or capsaicin contents. Although these vegetables have low-level toxic properties, they can contribute to various health problems over time.

Food vs. Medication

There will always be skeptics. The loudest argument heard so far about distrust for the diet approach in dealing with autoimmune diseases is: If immunosuppressive drugs are not completely effective in treating autoimmune diseases, how can diet do the magic? The diet approach is no magic - it is a scientific approach. Food is the key to health, wellness, and vitality. No pill can give as much antioxidants, vitamins, and other nutrients as fresh fruits and vegetables. Drugs are synthesized and are, therefore, not natural. Drugs riddle the body with side effects, whereas, food consumed in adequate amounts come with no side effects.

There are many reasons why the diet approach is safe and effective to repel the harm wrought by a malfunctioning immune system. The ultimate reason is that many foods have natural immunity-boost properties:

- A healthy digestive tract supports your immune system and food does this better than any pill;
- A serving of fruits is rich in natural micronutrients and phytonutrients that would unreasonably take dozens of synthetic supplement pills to match;
- Consumption of adequate protein and healthy fats strengthens your immune system way better than any immunosuppressive therapy can;
- Fiber-rich foods contain beta-glucan that helps the immune system defend the body from harmful substances like toxins, bacteria and viruses;
- Omega 3 fatty acids, together with omega 6 fatty acids, found in natural foods promote a two-pronged counter-attack against autoimmune diseases: a balanced immune system and a body better able to handle inflammation;
- Organic whole grains and protein sources act as natural defenders of the body against allergens and toxins that weaken the immune system;

- Nutrient-rich foods decrease your urge for calorie overload and prevent obesity. Medical evidence revealed that obesity weakens the body's immune functions.
- Mushrooms, among other foods, contain cytokines and polysaccharides that buttress the strength of the immune system;
- The more flavorful the spices are the more potent they are as immune boosters.

Food is potent medicine for autoimmune diseases and all diseases in general. Unlike the bitter pill, the cure that food offers for diseases is palatable. But in order for food to be able to perform its vaunted cure for many diseases, it has to be consumed in appropriate amounts.

The recipes in this book are prepared cautiously to come up with the most sumptuous meals that will help nourish and heal autoimmune diseases. They are easy to prepare and are sealed with natural curative ingredients from the best immunity-boosting foods. The diet approach to health is here. Get your kitchen busy and set your table ready for the revolutionary diet approach against autoimmune diseases. No more bitter pills to swallow!

SAMPLE RECIPES

Breakfast Ideas

Amazon Smoothie

Prep time: 5 minutes

INGREDIENTS

1 handful spinach

½ avocado

1 banana

1 large stalk celery

1 tsp cinnamon

1 cup water

INSTRUCTIONS

1. Slice avocado in half and remove the nut. Break the banana into small pieces and chop the celery into small pieces.
2. Combine all ingredients except for the spinach into a blender. Blend them until pureed, then add spinach and blend until pureed. Serve or chill and then serve.

Green Goodness Smoothie

Prep Time: 5 minutes

INGREDIENTS

2 cups spinach

2 whole kale leaves (1 cup chopped)

1 banana

1 green apple

1/2 cup green grapes

1 cup water (or fresh nut milk)

INSTRUCTIONS

1. Remove stems and ribs from kale. Core apple and dice. Peel banana.
2. Add water, banana and grapes to full sized blender. Process until solids are broken down.
3. Add greens and pulse on low for 30 seconds to break down. Then process on high for 1 minute, until smooth.
4. Pour into serving glasses and serve immediately.
5. Or chill in refrigerator for 20 minutes, blend for a few seconds to incorporate separated liquid, then pour into serving glasses and serve chilled.

Northern Typhoon

Prep time: 5 minutes

INGREDIENTS

1 handful Kale

1 banana

1 large cucumber

1 handful green beans

1 tsp cinnamon

1 cup water

INSTRUCTIONS

1. Break the banana into small pieces. De-stem the kale, skin and chop the cucumber and de-stem the green beans.

2. Combine all ingredients except for kale in a blender. Blend them until pureed, then add kale and blend until pureed. Serve or chill and then serve.

Pineapple Coconut Smoothie

Prep Time: 10 minutes*

INSTRUCTIONS

1 fresh coconut (or 1/2 cup flaked coconut)

1/2 cup pineapple chunks (fresh or frozen)

1 cup ice (crushed preferably)

Water

DIRECTIONS

1. *Soak flaked coconut in 1 1/2 cups water in refrigerator overnight, if using.
2. Add soaked coconut and soaking liquid to high-speed blender. Or remove flesh from fresh coconut and add to high-speed blender with 1 1/2 cups water. Process until well blended and fairly smooth, about 1 - 2 minutes.
3. Strain mixture through nut milk bag, cheesecloth or strainer back into blender.
4. Reserve pulp and set aside to dry and dehydrate, then use as coconut flour.
5. Cut pineapple flesh from peel, then chop. Add to blender with ice. Process until smooth, about 1 - 2 minutes.
6. Pour into serving glass and serve immediately.

Sweet Citrus Salad with Coconut Cream

Prep Time: 10 minutes

Servings: 1

INSTRUCTIONS

1 fresh coconut (or 1/2 cup flaked coconut)

1/4 - 1/3 cup dried pitted dates

1 blood orange

1 tangerine (or navel orange or clementine)

1/2 grapefruit (ruby red, pink or white)

1/2 lime

Water

INGREDIENTS

1. *Soak flaked coconut in 1 cup water overnight in refrigerator, if using. Soak dates in enough water to cover overnight in refrigerator. Drain.
2. Add soaked coconut and soaking liquid to high-speed blender. Or remove flesh from fresh coconut and add to high-speed blender with 3/4 cup water. Process until thick and fairly smooth, about 1 - 2 minutes.
3. Strain mixture through nut milk bag, cheesecloth or strainer back into blender or to food processor.
4. Reserve pulp and set aside to dry and dehydrate, then use as coconut flour.
5. Add soaked dates to processor and process until smooth. Set aside.

6. Peel all citrus and cut into segments. Add to serving dish. Top with sweet coconut cream.

7. Serve immediately. Or refrigerate 20 minutes and serve chilled.

Lunch and Dinner Ideas

Roasted Turkey Legs

Prep Time: 10 minutes*

Cook Time: 1 hour 20 minutes

Servings: 4

INGREDIENTS

2 large turkey legs

1/2 teaspoon garlic powder

1/2 teaspoon onion powder

1/2 teaspoon dried rosemary

1/2 teaspoon dried thyme

1/2 teaspoon Celtic sea salt

1 1/2 tablespoon coconut oil

Brine

4 cups water

1/4 cup Celtic sea salt

1/4 cup date butter

INSTRUCTIONS

1. *For *Brine*, add water, salt and date butter to wide, shallow container. Mix to combine. Add turkey legs and submerge completely in *Brine*. Marinate in refrigerator 12 - 24 hours.

2. Preheat oven to 350 degrees F. Place wire rack over sheet pan.

3. Remove turkey legs from brine. Rub salt, spices and oil over turkey legs, and under skin.

4. Place coated turkey legs on wire rack and bake about 35 - 40 minutes. Carefully turn turkey legs over and bake another 35 - 40 minutes, until skin is crisp and meat is cooked through.

5. Remove from oven and let rest about 2 minutes. Then serve hot.

Highland Beef Haggis

Prep Time: 10 minutes

Cook Time: 3 hours

Servings: 4

INGREDIENTS

8 oz (1/2 lb) ground beef (or bison, elk, etc.)

8 oz (1/2 lb) lamb shoulder

4 oz (1/4 lb) calves liver

2 onions (yellow or white)

1/2 head cauliflower (about 1 cup riced)

1 cup beef stock

2 garlic cloves

1/2 teaspoon ground nutmeg

1/4 teaspoon ground coriander

1/2 teaspoon Celtic sea salt

1/4 cup coconut oil

Water

INSTRUCTIONS

1. Preheat oven to 300 degrees F. Generously coat baking dish with coconut oil.
2. Add liver to small pan with enough water to cover over high heat. Bring to simmer and cook about 5 minutes. Drain and set aside to cool.

3. Roughly chop cauliflower. Peel and roughly chop onions and garlic. Add to food processor with lamb shoulder and par-cooked liver. Process until coarsely ground, about 2 minutes.

4. Add ground beef, stock, salt, and spices and pulse to combine. Transfer to prepared baking dish and cover tightly with aluminum foil.

5. Place covered dish in roasting pan. Add water to roasting pan 3/4 of the way up side of baking dish.

6. Bake for 3 hours. Remove from oven and carefully remove foil. Let rest about 10 minutes.

7. Remove baking dish from roasting pan. To plate, place serving dish over baking dish and carefully invert. Slice haggis into wedges and serve hot.

Bacon Wrapped Filet Mignon

Prep Time: 5 minutes

Cook Time: 20 minutes

Servings: 2

INGREDIENTS

2 (6 oz each) filet mignon steaks

2 thick slices nitrate-free bacon

Celtic sea salt, to taste

1 tablespoon coconut oil (optional)

Toothpicks

INSTRUCTIONS

1. Preheat oven to 350 degrees F. Heat medium oven-safe pan or skillet over medium heat.

2. Add bacon to hot pan. Cook and render out fat for about 5 minutes, until about halfway cooked. Remove bacon from pan and set aside, reserving bacon fat in pan. Add coconut oil to pan, if desired.

3. Wrap par-cooked bacon around steaks and secure with toothpick. Sprinkle steaks with salt to taste.

4. Add wrapped seasoned steaks to hot oiled pan and sear 2 minutes per side. Carefully flip half way through cooking.

5. Remove pan from stove and place in preheated oven. Cook about 8 - 10 minutes, until bacon is cooked through and steak is medium-rare.

6. Remove steaks from oven and transfer to cutting board. Set aside and let rest at least 2 minutes.

7. Transfer to serving dish and serve hot.

Herb Roasted Pork Tenderloin

Prep Time: 10 minutes*

Cook Time: 15 minutes

Servings: 4

INGREDIENTS

1 pork tenderloin

1 teaspoon dried rosemary

1 teaspoon dried thyme

1 teaspoon dried oregano

1 teaspoon dried basil

1 teaspoon dried marjoram (optional)

1 teaspoon Celtic sea salt

Apricot Sauce

1 cup dried apricots

2/3 cup water

1 teaspoon apple cider vinegar (or dry white wine)

INSTRUCTIONS

1. Preheat oven to 425 degrees F. Heat small pan over medium heat.
2. Rub tenderloin with salt and spices, then press into meat so it adheres. Place on sheet pan, or wire rack over sheet pan.
3. Roast for 10 - 15 minutes, until just cooked through and no pink remains. Remove pork from oven and let rest 10 minutes.

4. For *Apricot Sauce*, add dried apricots, water and vinegar to food processor or high-speed blender. Process until smooth, about 1 - 2 minutes.

5. Add *Apricot Sauce* to hot pan and reduce until slightly thickened. Stir well and do not let burn. Remove from heat.

6. Slice pork and transfer to serving dish. Top pork with *Apricot Sauce* and serve warm.

Classic Churrasco with Chimichurri

Prep Time: 10 minutes*

Cook Time: 5 minutes

Servings: 4

INGREDIENTS

24 oz (1 1/2 lb) beef tenderloin

Chimichurri

1 cup coconut oil

1/3 cup apple cider vinegar (or coconut aminos)

1/3 cup water

1 large bunch cilantro

1 large bunch parsley

1/2 cup fresh mint leaves

6 garlic cloves

1 teaspoon Celtic sea salt

INSTRUCTIONS

1. For *Chimichurri*, peel garlic and add to food processor or high-speed blender. Remove cilantro, parsley and mint leaves from stems. Add to processor and process to finely chop, about 1 minute. Add oil, water, salt and spices. Process until thick sauce forms, about 1 - 2 minutes.

2. Cut tenderloin lengthwise into 4 even slices, then flatten with tenderizing or kitchen mallet to 1/2 inch thickness. Place meat in between two parchment sheets to flatten, if preferred.

3. *Pour 1/4 of the *Chimichurri* into a baking dish just large enough to fit tenderloin. Place beef over *Chimichurri*, then top with second 1/4 of *Chimichurri*. Set aside to marinate about 1 hour. Transfer remaining *Chimichurri* to serving dish.

4. Heat grill or grated skillet over high heat.

Moist Roasted Turkey

Prep Time: 10 minutes*

Cook Time: 4 - 6 hours

Servings: 12

INGREDIENTS

20 lb (approx.) whole turkey

2 teaspoons Celtic sea salt

2 tablespoons coconut oil

Brine

1 - 2 gallons water

1 cup Celtic sea salt

1 cup date butter

INSTRUCTIONS

1. *For *Brine*, add 1/2 gallon of water, salt and date butter to large baking dish or roasting pan. Mix to combine. Remove any entrails from turkey and add to *Brine*, plus and enough water to submerge completely. Marinate in refrigerator 12 - 24 hours.

2. Preheat oven to 350 degrees F. Place roasting rack in clean roasting pan.

3. Drain turkey and rub salt and oil over and under skin, where possible.

4. Place seasoned turkey on roasting rack and bake about 15 - 18 minutes per lb, about 5 hours for 20 lb bird. Or until internal

temperature reaches 165 degrees F. Baste with rendered fat and juices throughout cooking for even browning.

5. Remove turkey from oven and let rest 20 - 30 minutes.
6. Carve and serve warm.

Quick Raw Avocado Slaw

Prep Time: 10 minutes*

Cook Time: 20 minutes

Servings: 4

INGREDIENTS

1/2 head cabbage (2 cups shredded)

1 avocado

1 carrot

Zest of 1 lemon

Juice of 1 lemon

1 tablespoon raw honey

2 tablespoons apple cider vinegar

1 teaspoon sea salt

INSTRUCTIONS

1. Cut avocado in half and remove pit. Scoop flesh into large mixing bowl and mash with fork.
2. Remove any tough outer leaves and core from cabbage. Shred cabbage and carrot. Add to bowl with vinegar, honey and salt. Zest *then* juice lemon, and add.
3. Toss to combine.
4. Serve immediately. Or and place in refrigerator for 20 minutes and serve chilled.

Snack Ideas

Smoked Salmon and Avocado Snack

Prep Time: 5* minutes

Servings: 2

INGREDIENTS

4 oz (1 or 1/2 package) cold-smoked salmon

1 avocado

1 stalk fresh dill

Pinch sea salt

1/2 lemon (optional)

INSTRUCTIONS

1. Slice avocado in half and remove pit. Cut into thick slices in peel then scoop out with large spoon.
2. Slice smoked salmon into long 1 inch strips. Wrap 1 salmon strips around each avocado slice. Arrange wrapped avocado on serving dish.
3. Mince fresh dill. Sprinkle dill and salt over avocado wraps and serve immediately.
4. Or squeeze juice of 1/2 lemon over avocado wraps, sprinkle on dill and salt, and refrigerate 20 minutes. Then serve chilled.

Olive Tapenade

Prep Time: 15 minutes

Servings: 2

INGREDIENTS

1 1/2 cups any combination pitted olives (Kalamata, Spanish, black, pimento, etc.)

2 tablespoons capers

2 anchovy fillets

1 garlic clove

2 fresh basil leaves

1/2 lemon

2 tablespoons coconut oil

INSTRUCTIONS

1. Peel garlic and add to food processor or high-speed blender. Process until finely ground.
2. Rinse and drain olives, capers and anchovy fillets. Add to processor with basil, oil and squeeze of 1/2 lemon. Process until finely chopped or coarsely ground, about 1 - 2 minutes.
3. Transfer to serving dish and serve immediately.

Spicy Tuna Tartare

Prep Time: 15* minutes

Servings: 4

INGREDIENTS

1 lb tuna steak (sushi grade)

1 small cucumber

1 ripe avocado

1 lime

1 garlic clove

2 tablespoons raw virgin coconut oil

Small bunch fresh cilantro

1 teaspoon sea salt

INSTRUCTIONS

1. Peel, seed and dice cucumber and avocado. Finely chop cilantro. Add to medium mixing bowl.
2. Remove seeds, stem and veins from hot pepper. Peel garlic and add to food processor or bullet blender. Process until smooth paste forms. Add to bowl.
3. Dice tuna, discarding any tough white gristle. Add to bowl.
4. Squeeze on lime juice and add salt.
5. Gently toss with soft spatula or large spoon.
6. Serve immediately. Or refrigerate 20 minutes and serve chilled.

Baked Candied Yams

Prep Time: 10 minutes

Cook Time: 1 hour 30 minutes

Servings: 12

INGREDIENTS

4 large sweet potatoes (yams)

1/2 cup dried pitted dates

1/4 cup dried apricots

2 tablespoons coconut butter

1 tablespoon ground cinnamon

1/2 teaspoon ground ginger

Pinch Celtic sea salt

Topping

1/4 cup date butter

INSTRUCTIONS

1. Preheat oven to 350 degrees F.
2. Gently rinse sweet potatoes and place on sheet pan.
3. Bake about 1 hour, until tender.
4. Add dates, apricots and enough water to cover in small pot. Heat over medium heat. Let simmer until water evaporates. Remove from heat.
5. Remove yams from oven and let cool about 10 minutes.

6. For *Topping*, add date butter to small pan. Heat over medium heat and cook for about 4 - 5 minutes. Stir frequently and do not burn. Remove from heat and set aside.

7. Add softened dates and apricots to large mixing bowl. Mash with potato masher, hand mixer or whisk.

8. Cut yams open lengthwise and scoop flesh into mixing bowl. Add butter, salt and spices. Mash with potato masher, hand mixer or whisk until well combined.

9. Transfer yam mixture to serving dish and top with *Topping*. Serve warm.

Lean Mean Collard Greens

Prep Time: 15 minutes

Cook Time: 2 1/2 hours

Servings: 8

INGREDIENTS

2 heads (or 2 large bags) fresh collard greens

6 slices nitrate-free bacon (or 1 small ham hock)

8 cups chicken stock

Water

INSTRUCTIONS

1. Preheat oven to 350 degrees F. Heat large pot over medium-high heat.
2. Rinse collards well and roughly chop. Place in large colander or in clean sink to drain.
3. Add bacon or ham hock to hot pot and render down for about 5 minutes.
4. Add greens to pot in batches. If all greens to not fit, reserve. Add chicken stock.
5. Bring pot to a simmer then reduce to low heat. Add any remaining greens, plus enough water just to cover, if necessary. Stir gently.
6. Simmer until collards are tender, about 2 - 2 1/2 hours.
7. Drain greens well. Transfer to serving dish and serve warm.

5. Place beef on grill or skillet on the diagonal and cook for about 1 minute, then rotate meat to create crosshatch grill marks and cook

for another minute. Then flip and repeat. Cook for about 4 minutes total for medium rare.

6. Remove from grill, slice against the grain and transfer to serving dish. Serve immediately with *Chimichurri*.

Turkey Jerky Bacon

Prep Time: 10 minutes*

Dehydrating Time: 4 - 8 hours

Servings: 4

INGREDIENTS

4 oz organic turkey (dark meat)

2 tablespoons coconut aminos (or liquid aminos)

2 tablespoons tamari (or liquid aminos or coconut aminos)

1 tablespoon lemon juice (or raw apple cider vinegar)

1 tablespoons Celtic sea salt

1/2 teaspoon garlic powder

1/2 teaspoon onion powder

INSTRUCTIONS

1. Prepare two sheet parchment. Lay one on cutting board.

2. Cut turkey into 1/4 inch strips and lay in single layer on parchment. Pound with tenderizing side of kitchen mallet. Cover turkey with second parchment sheet, then pound with flat side of tenderizing mallet to 1/8 inch thickness.

3. *Place turkey strips in medium mixing bowl or shallow dish. Add coconut aminos, tamari, lemon juice, salt and spices. Mix well to coat. Cover and place in refrigerator for 8 hours, or overnight.

4. Remove turkey from refrigerator and lay in single layer on dehydrator trays. Place trays in dehydrator and set to 120 degrees F for 4 - 8 hours.

5. After 4 hours dehydrating time, remove trays from dehydrator and test turkey by bending. If it cracks, remove and serve immediately. Or store in airtight container.

6. If still flexible, place back in dehydrator and continue dehydrating up to 4 hours, or until desired texture is achieved.

www.ingramcontent.com/pod-product-compliance
Lightning Source LLC
Chambersburg PA
CBHW070130290526
45789CB00005B/2184